# My Nepenthe

## Chapter 1

### The Call

Chaplain: I'm so very sorry to be meeting you under these circumstances. Can you tell me a little bit about what the doctors have said to you this morning?

Mother: "They said she was hit by a car near school and to prepare ourselves that she may not make it. Her GCS is only a three and it needs to get higher so that we can all go home. Why do I need to prepare myself for the worst? Look...she is still breathing! Look at those machines! I see the monitors with a heart beat and she has a blood pressure as well! Help me understand what you are saying simply... What is this GCS brain flow test? Did she fail? This makes no sense at all."

Chaplain: I will try to explain this to you as simply as possible. Thereare two ways a person can die. The first way we can all recognize quickly. The heart stops, and the patient flat-lines with no pulse or heart beat. We shock the heart in hopes of resuscitation. And if it works we regain a pulse and the heart then beats in a steady rhythm. Each heartbeat gives us hope for more life.

The heart can stop and that is the first way. But remember there are two ways a person can die...yet the other one is rarely talked about.

The second way a person can die is brain death. This is confusing and tricky for those hoping and praying for their loved ones. Traumatized families are often given a grave prognosis and do not realize what the physicians are actually telling them. Their loved ones may have been in an accident, had a traumatic brain injury or a brain aneurism.

Their loved one still seems to be breathing, the heartbeat is still there, the chest is moving up and down and the skin is still pink and warm.

But brain death is real death. It is irreversible. It cannot be recovered from. The brain cannot be reset.

Imagine the brain is like a light bulb. When healthy and active thereis activity within the top of the bulb (Chaplain makes hands in the shape of the bulb with tapping fingers moving quickly inside the bulb). A person who has died from brain death has no activity in their bulb. (The chaplain looks through empty hands right into the eyes of the mother of the patient.)

The hospital tested your daughter with the CBF or a cerebral bloodflow test...cerebral meaning brain. So it's a brain blood-flow test. And this test showed no blood flow to her brain. No blood flow to her brain or no activity within her light bulb.

The CBF test proves there is no blood flow or activity into those areas of her brain that control her body or her responses. The GCS Number has a range of 3 to 15, or Glasgow Coma Scale. Right now, you and I talking here together, we both have an average GCS above 15. Your daughter has a GCS of 3. That is the lowest number! So I will explain how they arrived at the GCS of 3.

You would never allow me to poke you in your eye with my fingers, or put my fingers down your throat. You would certainly respond if I pricked your toe with a sharp pin or if I put ice-cold water into your ear. A lower GCS number indicates that a person has little or no response to these types of tests. There is no response with the voice or eyes or by even moving the body.

Your daughter had no response to any of the tests. In fact, themovement you see in her body right now is happening only because of the machines attached to her body. It is moving the blood and oxygen through

her body. The machines are the reason her chest is rising and falling. The machines are keeping her heartbeat and blood pressure going by providing mechanical support to her organs.

If we remove all of the machines, the blood and oxygen will stop moving and your daughter will not breathe on her own. They showed this to you in the apnea test this morning. Remember that she did not ever breathe on her own for over ten minutes.

I understand this confusion. If it were my

daughter on that bed I would want to understand how they really knew that my child was brain dead.

Your daughter has no blood flow to her brain. She can not breathe or move the blood and oxygen on her own. She has no responses in any way. And brain death is death. It cannot be reversed. It cannot be recovered from. Unlike the heart, there is no way to restart the brain.

Brain death is death and unfortunately your daughter died today at 11:15 am. Her clinical time of death was recorded today at 11:15 am. And if it is okay with you I would like to talk with you about the next steps in the process.

Your family is in a very unique situation with your daughter's death to give the gift of life to another person, several people in fact, through organ donation.

Most people understand as little about organ donation as they do about brain death. The truth is that there are families on other floors of this hospital praying that their loved ones will receive healing through their last hope.....that someone like your daughter will donate her organs. They are the most ill patients that are waiting on the UNOS list.

Your daughter has the unique ability in her final hours to give many other people a lifetime. As an organ donor your daughter may give her heart, lungs, liver, pancreas, intestines and kidneys. Several of her life-saving vital organs, the kidneys and the lungs, may be divided and shared with up to 4 recipients. She could also give the gift of sight to a blind person through cornea donation.

And to be a little bit graphic for a minute...cornea donation is not the same thing as eyeball donation. They take just the tiny corneas from the donor. They are thinner than a contact lens. Corneal transplant surgery is the only known cure for vision loss or blindness.

Every gift is procured in this hospital with the same respectfulsurgical procedures and integrity that we provide during any transplant surgery. In fact the transplant teams will assemble here at this hospital to recover these gifts.

In her final hours your daughter really can give another person a lifetime. We would start by keeping her connected to the machines and transport her to the operating room where transplant teams would be standing by to recover the gifts.

Today in this hospital those transplant teams are here for living organ donors or those who are voluntarily giving a kidney, a lung, or a portion of their livers, to another gravely-ill person. The gifts may be given to a complete stranger or to a dearly beloved family member waiting on the UNOS Transplant List. Either way they are giving the gift of life to another human being... and I can think of no greater love.

Mother: I think we would like to donate her organs. Can we know who gets them?

Father: We both know that it is what she would have wanted to do.

Chaplains: To answer your questions, yes, there is a means of communication set up which allows recipients and donors to communicate and exchange letters. The recipients and their families understand the gravity of the life-saving gifts that they received from the donors. They often have letters prepared in advance as they fight for their lives while waiting on the UNOS registry.

If both parties express a desire to meet and communicate further we help to make that happen. So the simple answer is yes.... if that is what both parties wish to happen.

As far as deciding who receives the gifts, the primary match happensby blood-type and tissue-type matching followed by other medical factors.

The transplant team operates from the national UNOS database. There are over 100,000 people waiting on the transplant list. Each giftis offered to the transplant team of the best-matched patient. The sickest patient receives the gift.

Mother: Ok, but what about her funeral? Can we still have an open casket at her funeral?

Chaplain: That is a great question and the

answer is yes. Many of our donor families have open-casket funerals after their loved ones have given the gift of life through organ donation. Again, the same respectful surgical procedures are performed here in the hospital by highly-trained transplant surgeons.

After the recovery of the gifts, the bodies are then released to the Medical Examiners' office and then finally to the funeral home of your choice. Organ donors have funerals and memorial services just like any of the other patients who die in this hospital. However, I do think that there is one significant difference between your daughter and most other people who die in this hospital: I don't know many heroes in real life myself.... but I do believe that by giving the gift of life to another person, your daughter would be a real hero.

## Chapter 2

## NOT YOUR TYPICAL SILVER LINING

Chaplain: I'm sorry to be meeting your family under thesecircumstances. This is a conversation that no one wants to have....ever. The decision for compassionate withdrawal of life support is never a simple one. Can you tell me what you understand has happened toyour brother?

Sister: My brother is a good man deep down. He has been strugglingwith depression for the last three years since his wife's death. Icannot believe that he would do this to himself. His daughter, my niece, found him hanging in the garage. They say that he has permanent brain damage because of the lack of oxygen to his brain. My niece cut him down as quickly as she could but they say it was too late. They just finished doing all of the tests on his brain. His brain is not working enough and it will never work again. He is basically gone. He is barely breathing and he was shocked with those heart paddles twice already this morning. Ugh, Oh God! I need to call his work and tell them he is in the hospital. Where is my phone?

Chaplain: Here, you can use my phone or I can ask the nurse to help us make the calls. If you prefer, I can sit here with you while you make the calls.

Nurse: We informed his work in the Emergency Department with his Insurance Card information. They are aware that he is here.

Chaplain: Speaking of calls, is there someone from your faith practice that I can contact to join us here as we walk through the next steps in this process?

Sister: No. Not with this kind of thing.....especially when they find out it wasn't an accident. They are probably going to think that he is a goingto hell. I don't want this to be the only thing people remember about him or his life.

Chaplain: I believe that most people, from a church or not, would see this situation as a person who was in a lot of pain. He was already living in a hell of pain and suffering. People who complete suicide are often looking for a way to stop their pain and see no other way out. And for the record, no one deserves to have their whole life judged or defined by one choice that they make. We can't know the last things that he thought, or did, or might have prayed. And this doesn't have to be the last chapter of

his legacy.Sister: No? How do you figure that?

Chaplain: No, He can give the gift of life through organ donation after the compassionate withdrawal of life support. He could give life-saving organs such as his liver or his kidneys and save the lives of others. This does not have to be the ending to his story.

Sister: Even if I sign the papers to take away the machines and let him go in peace, he can still help or save other people?

Chaplain: Yes, organs remain healthy only for a short period of time after the removal of the mechanical support, so every minute counts... but yes. We can work together to make a plan to provide a meaningful goodbye to your brother as we let him go in peace and enable his legacy to live on.

Sister: My father-in-law needs a kidney transplant but we didn't wantto bother my brother to test his blood because he was feeling so down lately. And now that we are talking about this, I remember my brother saying he would let them have anything if it could help someone else. He told me that once before. It was back when he got his driver's license. He said that he signed up to be an organ donor at the DMV. It is exactly what he said he wanted to do. I am just surprised that we can still do this for him now.

Chaplain: If your brother and your father-in-law are a positive matchyou can then participate in what is known as direct donation. And of course he can help others waiting for life-saving transplants with his other gifts.

Your brother would be giving a legacy of life in his death. Your brother's legacy will forever be that he gave the gift of life. He will live on through them.

## Chapter 3

## NEVER RIGHT

Chaplain: I'm sorry to be meeting your family under these circumstances. This is a conversation that no parent ever wants to have. Can you tell me what the doctors have explained to you about your son?

Mother: They say he has a problem with his head and his eyes. I don't know how it happened but he must have fallen from his crib. He has been teething and crying all the time. Maybe he has a toothache or something. They say that he has a detached retina. The police have asked me what happened to him, but I was at work all day. He was with my boyfriend. When I came in from work the baby was too still. He was just lying there kind of limp. He must have fallen and hit his head somewhere but he doesn't have any broken bones that I could see. We have been here waiting for them to tell us what's really wrong with him. They took my boyfriend out to talk to him about what happened a while ago. He was very upset and crying over my son by the hospital bed. But Itold them everything I know.

Chaplain: Is your son's biological father here too?

Mother: No, he doesn't claim my son as his anyways. They said they were calling him to tell him to get down here. He has threatened my boyfriend a bunch of times. He needs to leave us alone. The doctors said thatthey were doing everything that they could to help my son.

Chaplain: So he is on his way to the hospital then? Mother: I don't know.

Chaplain: When he gets here we can talk with you both about the next steps in this process.

Mother: I can hear my boyfriend calling for me so I need to go. Chaplain: OK we can talk in a little while then.Mother: I already told you everything that I know.Chaplain: Yes, you already told me what you know.

Nurse: Chaplain, Can you please come over to our private consult room? Chaplain: Of course.

Nurse: The child has severe brain swelling and a detached retina. The child has extensive older fractures visible on his x-rays. All tests conclusively show that the child was violently shaken and received trauma to the base of his skull.

The mother now refuses to give any additional information to our team. I think she is trying to protect her boyfriend. He was the one who was screaming down the hallway for her to get the child's father out of his sight.

Chaplain: So the child's father is here now?

Nurse: Yes. He threatened to throw the boyfriend out the window. This is a total circus. We have both security and the police here now.Child protective services are en route. Clinically speaking, the child has a GCS of 3 and has no spontaneous responses whatsoever. They conducted the apnea test earlier. The apnea test showed the child had no spontaneous breathing. Radiology has returned the CBF results for the second neurologist's note and it shows no cerebral blood flow to the brain. The child has been declared brain dead and the clinical time of death was given when the second neurologist signed his note.

The physicians consulted with both the parents a while ago to give them the grave prognosis. We put both parents in the large family respite room so that you can speak with the mother and father privately.

And just so you know, they are very angry.

I do not envy you, Chaplain. I'm sure that this will be a very challenging conversation.

Chaplain: OK, Thank you for letting me know.

--- In the family respite room---

Father: Now what is this about? They couldn't help save my son. Now what do you want? You know they didn't help him as much as they could have .....because we don't ever get the same kind of help that you all do. I don't trust any of you all. This ain't right and it will never be right.

Chaplain: You are correct in that this will never be right. It goes completely against the natural order of things. Children should always outlive their parents. I agree. A parent who has to outlive his or her own child... that could never be right.

No parent wants to have this kind of conversation but you two have the ability to help other children who are dying in children's hospitals like this one...tonight. It is within your power to help other parents to NOT have the conversations like the ones you both have had today. Your son has the ability to give the gift of life to several children by giving them the gift of life through organ donation.

Father: It's probably the same people who let him die that now want to sell his body parts to the people who got money.

Chaplain: Every physician in this facility has made it their life's work to save as many children as possible. Even though the medical team members do everything they can to save a patient's life, sometimes the injuries are too severe and the patient dies. If the patient is not responding, physicians will then perform a series of tests to determine if brain death has occurred. A patient who is brain dead has no brain activity and cannot breathe on his or her own. Brain death is death and it is irreversible. Someone who is brain dead cannot recover. ONLY AFTER brain death has been confirmed and the time of death noted, only then can organ donation even become a possibility.

Donation of organs and tissues takes place

only after all lifesaving efforts have been exhausted, death has been legally declared, and donor designation has been confirmed. If an individual like your son cannot or did not previously designate his wishes, the next-of-kin would then have to give consent before donation could take place. You, his parents, are the only ones who can give that consent.

African Americans, Hispanics and other minorities are more than half of those patients awaiting lifesaving organ transplants. That is because there is a greater prevalence of some illnesses, including kidney disease, within these communities.

As a matter of fact, African Americans and Hispanics are three times more likely to suffer from end-stage renal disease. Although donors and recipients do not have to share the same ethnicity, transplant success increases when organs are matched between donors and recipients of the same ethnic background. Unfortunately, the lack of organs donated from multicultural populations can contribute to longer waiting periods for patients in need of transplants. Many patients do not receive a transplant in time. The UNOS wait list gives no special treatment. The sickest patient on the UNOS list always receives the organs unless the donor family has opted for direct donation to their own loved ones or to a person that they designate. The sickest children on the transplant wait list would be the ones to receive the gifts of life from your son.

In his death, he could save a child who needs a heart, another who needs lungs to breathe, and another who needs a life-saving liver or pancreas transplant to survive and thrive. Seven or eight lives may be saved. Many parents just like you are hoping and praying that their child won't die tonight. Those kids can be given the gift of life from your child in his death.

And finally, there is no cost for donation. The donor family is not responsible for any fees associated with donation. Ever.

You are right....this will never be right....kids shouldn't die beforetheir parents. But it is in your power... the both of you... to help to save these kids.

Father: We can still help make it right for those kids even though he is dead?

Chaplain: YES. In his final hour he can still give them a lifetime. Father: Help those kids.Mother: Yes, we have to try to make this right.

## Chapter 4

## FAITH FOR MORE

Chaplain: I'm sorry to be meeting you under these circumstances. Can you tell me what the doctors have explained to you about your wife?

Husband: She just delivered our newborn son four days ago. When we got back home she said that she had a headache and wanted to lie down for a little while. She lay down on our bed and she never really wokeup. They said that she had a massive brain aneurism. I have been here for two days and she is only getting worse every hour. They said she has no blood flow to her brain, that she won't breathe on her own and that she does not respond to any treatment. The doctors told me today thatshe might going for good. But I told them that I believe in miracles and that God could still heal her if He wanted to!

Chaplain: I absolutely believe in miracles too. God can provide miracles in the most unexpected ways. Even when they are not the miracles that we were hoping or praying for, other miracles can still unfold! Your wife now has the ability to be the miracle by giving the gift of life to others through organ donation.

Husband: She was a good person and she would give the shirt off her back to help anyone. She would want to help people. How can she help people?

Chaplain: Heart and lung transplants allow people to survive and thrive.

Kidney transplantation allows the recipient to live a life free from dialysis treatments. Pancreas transplantation releases the diabetic from insulin therapy and halts the progress of a ravaging disease.Liver transplantation saves the lives of many children as well as adults. Our livers must function for our bodies to survive and thrive.

Life-enhancing gifts like cornea transplants let people see the beauty of the world around them. A cornea transplant can literally make the blind see. Intestinal transplants let the recipients receive life-sustaining nutrients and energy from food instead of tubes. Heart valves save the lives of those threatened by heart disease or malfunction. And there are so many more.

Most major religions consider organ donation as one of the greatest expressions of compassion and generosity. It can provide families with a sense that their loved one will live on and that something good has come from a very bad situation.

Husband: This is what she would want and this is what we are going to do. We will be the miracle.

## Chapter 5

## UNTIL WE GET HOME

Chaplain: I'm so very sorry to be meeting you under these circumstances but I understand that you have asked to speak with me.

Father: Yes, my wife is a registered organ donor and she is also brain dead. I know exactly what this means because we both registered to be organ donors together. I just cannot think of a way to tell my children about what has happened, what will happen to her and what this all really means. We have 5 young children under the age of 11. Our pastor is in the waiting room with our kids but I understand that you know a way to tell them and that you were trained to do this type of thing. Please, can you help us?

Chaplain: I am absolutely willing to do whatever I can to help you and your children during this difficult time. You mentioned your pastor was here? What faith practice is your family a part of?

Father: Agape, it's a nondenominational Christian church. Our family believes in God, the Bible and in Prayer. One of our kids' Sunday School teachers is also with them in the waiting room.

Chaplain: OK. That information will help me frame the words that I use when I speak with them as a group. It is important that we use honest and age-appropriate language when we explain these things to children. If we simply say they have gone to sleep, many kids become fearful of ever falling asleep again. We shouldn't say that they have gone to the light because kids have asked me when will they turn the lights off and let my mommy come back home? Honest and age-appropriate language is critical.... and so is not scaring them. It will also help me if you will explain to me what your family believes happens when we die. Do you believe in heaven as it is described in the Bible as you mentioned? Is this what your children have been taught too?

Father: Yes, we believe in heaven like it says in the Bible. The kids believe it too. We have been talking even more about our faith recently since it's so close to the holidays.

Chaplain: Okay that will help me explain the context to them. I will get down at their eye level and make sure that I slowly explain what has happened and why their mommy is a real life hero who helps God with miracles.

--- In A Private Family Waiting Room ---

Chaplain: I was hoping that I would have a chance to meet all five of you. I know that you have all been waiting a very long time. At least up here on this floor, with the good windows, we can see what is going on outside. I was curious do any of you know where heaven is?

Child 1- It is up there in the big blue sky.

Chaplain: That is right! Wow, you are really smart. Do you know who lives there in heaven?

Child 2 & Child 3 (overlapping): God, Jesus, big angels, our other brown dog, grandpa.

Chaplain: Yes that is right. All of them are in heaven. So you allknow that we all lived in heaven first because the Bible says that God created heaven and the earth. It also says that God knew every one of us when we were inside our mommies' tummies. God knew us before we were born when we lived in heaven with Him. Then we were born and came to live here for a little while, and one day we will go back home to heaven to all be together again. Jesus said that He would make a place for us in heaven and when it was our time to go home He would be waiting there for us too. Did you say that your grandpa is there in heaven too? Did he die?

Oldest Child: Yes, he died at the start of the school year.

Child 4: He was an army captain and they fired guns at the cemetery that were really loud. My grandma said don't be too sad though because he was in heaven with God.

Chaplain: Yes, I see. It is really hard to let people go back home to heaven because we always miss them so much here, don't we? The reason I came in here was to tell you all that your mommy has been making her trip back home to heaven today. She has gone back home to heaven because she died too. She died today and has gone back home to be in heaven. I am very sorry that she died. It is okay to be very sad but it is nice that your grandpa will be waiting for her in heaven when she gets back home. When she is in heaven I'm sure she will talk with your grandpa about what it feels like being a hero. Your grandpa helped save people's lives when he was in the war and your mommy helped to save people's lives by helping them when they were really sick. Mommies always help us feel better when we are sick, don't they?

Well, like I said, I am very, very sorry that your mommy died and it really is okay to be sad and to miss her. If you want to you can always talk to her up in heaven any time you want to because heaven makes her ears really, really strong. And then one day a very long time from now we will go back home to heaven too and we will all be together again. And that makes me happy because I sometimes miss those in my family who have already gone home too.

**Chapter 6**

**A PART OF ME**

Man: Hi Chaplain, Do you remember me? About 3 years ago my wife and older son were in a tragic car accident along with my younger son. My younger son was the only one who survived the accident.

Chaplain: Yes, of course I remember you and I remember your family. I hope you're not here at the hospital for your family again today.

Man: No, not exactly. It's a little bit of a crazy story but so special that I just had to come and tell you about it. As you know, I really struggled with the decision to withdraw my late wife's life support. Our older son was DOA when they brought them both here to the hospital after the accident. We couldn't do anything to help him so it felt like I should do everything I could to help my wife at that time. I resisted everything and everyone. You know.....you were there!

Well I sat beside my wife's hospital bed and watched her vitals on the monitors and machines. They slowly kept going from bad to worse! Her vitals were going and I knew that I needed to let her go, but I just couldn't. I told her she couldn't leave me alone without her help to raise our younger son. I cried and begged her. I begged God to let me keep her! I needed something to help me with our son who survived. I was terrified of how I would do it all alone.

Of course you know that finally we let her go peacefully, and she donated her gifts. I decided that she would give her gifts after we withdrewthe machines and that's exactly what she did. Her kidneys went totwo different recipients, her heart valves helped another young mom, her corneas gave a college kid his vision back. That guy keeps an Instagram account in my wife's honor and says that the world is so much more beautiful through her eyes!

Having contact with the people whose lives were changed by my late wife's gifts really helped both me and my son in the early days of our grief. Oh and her liver.... her liver is the reason that I am actually here today. About eight months after my wife passed I received a letter through the Transplant team's office. The letter was from the person who receivedmy late wife's liver. The letter told me so much about the struggle to survive with a malfunctioning liver. We began to write letters and finally we decided to talk to one another in person.

I know this sounds crazy but the person that received my wife's liver is now my fiancé! We just got engaged over the holidays! So my wife really saved a part of herself to help me with our younger son after all! His soon-to-be step-mom has a part of his birth-mom too. God must have been listening to my prayers after all.

Chaplain: Wow! That is truly an incredible story!!! After hearing your story, I know that my prayers were answered too! Thank you for sharing it with me! May God Bless you in your new beginning! Now your future sacredly holds a piece of your past too!

www.ingramcontent.com/pod-product-compliance
Lightning Source LLC
Chambersburg PA
CBHW072306170526
45158CB00003BA/1204